How to Have a

MINDFUL
PREGNANCY
& BIRTH

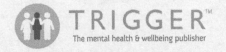

The mental health & wellbeing publisher

PRAISE FOR THIS BOOK

ABOUT THE AUTHORS

Dr Sian Warriner RM, MSc, DClinPrac is a consultant midwife and mother of four boys. She leads the Mindfulness-Based Childbirth and Parenting antenatal education programme for the Oxford University Hospitals NHS Foundation Trust, and is a teaching partner at the Oxford Mindfulness Centre, University of Oxford. She is lead author of the study 'An Evaluation of Mindfulness-Based Childbirth and Parenting Courses for Pregnant Women and Prospective Fathers/Partners within the UK NHS' (Midwifery, 2018).

Mark Pallis has two young children and is the author of several books, including the popular mindful storytime book for children, *Crab and Whale* (Mindful Storytime Press, 2018).

How to Have a

MINDFUL PREGNANCY & BIRTH

30 Simple Ways to Connect With Your Baby and Your Body

SIAN WARRINER
AND MARK PALLIS

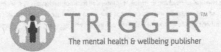
TRIGGER™
The mental health & wellbeing publisher

This edition published in 2023 by Trigger Publishing
An imprint of Shaw Callaghan Ltd

UK Office
The Stanley Building
7 Pancras Square
Kings Cross
London N1C 4AG

US Office
On Point Executive Center, Inc
3030 N Rocky Point Drive W
Suite 150
Tampa, FL 33607
www.triggerhub.org

Text Copyright © 2021 Sian Warriner and Mark Pallis
First published in 2021 by Welbeck Balance

A CIP catalogue record for this book is available upon request from the British Library
ISBN: 978-1-83796-252-5
Ebook ISBN: 978-1-83796-253-2

Typeset by stevewilliamscreative.com

For the women who have taught me, my
MBCP friends and colleagues. SW

For Benedetta with love. MP

CONTENTS

CONTENTS

CHAPTER 2

A Time to Enjoy and be Proud of Your Pregnancy

CHAPTER 3

A Time to Slow Down and Nurture Yourself

CHAPTER 6

PARENTHOOD: A New Way of Being ....

INTRODUCTION TO MINDFULNESS

JUST AS YOU ARE

By Sian Warriner

Hi, I'm Sian and I have had the privilege of working as a midwife for over 30 years, helping to support women and their families through pregnancy and birth.

A wise colleague once described the joys and challenges of pregnancy and birth to me as transformational: a moment in time when our lives change forever. She was right. The occasion of pregnancy, birth and becoming a parent is often a time when we take stock and choose to make intentional, positive changes – and mindfulness can be incredibly helpful with this.

This book offers 30 simple ways that you, as a mum-to-be who still has to navigate day-to-day life, can start to bring mindfulness into your pregnancy and beyond, just as you are – whether or not you've ever tried mindfulness before.

Why Mindfulness?

Mindfulness is the practice of bringing your attention to whatever is happening in the present moment. As you will see later in the book, this can be your breath, the sensations in your body (experienced through your five senses), your everyday actions (such as brushing your teeth or going for a walk), or your emotions ... almost anything in fact. The key is to *intentionally* experience the present moment, with kindness, with self-compassion and without judging yourself – just being *in* the moment as best you can.

Over the past two decades, the practice of mindfulness has evolved from its Eastern meditation roots to a mainstream, secular and increasingly accessible way of supporting our mental health and emotional wellbeing. We now have strong, scientifically robust evidence that a regular mindfulness practice can shift us from a place where we may feel overwhelmed, stressed or out of control to a calmer and more contented headspace.

Everyone's experience of pregnancy is different. Nevertheless, I've seen first-hand how mindfulness can provide the tools to help women more smoothly navigate the wonderful-yet-demanding time that is pregnancy and the birth of their baby. Rather than simply "getting through" this time, with mindfulness mums-to-be can thrive and become fully present for all the inevitable ups and downs that it holds. Learning the art of mindfulness will give you a set of simple yet hugely powerful skills that can completely transform your emotional experience and sense of wellbeing.

Does Mindfulness Actually Help During Pregnancy?

The short answer is "yes".

In 2018, I led a research team studying the effects of mindfulness in pregnancy, birth and into parenthood (Warriner *et al*, 2018). Our study showed that using mindfulness techniques in pregnancy really can reduce pregnancy-related worry and allow more space for life to be "just as it is" – and that this builds self-compassion and inner calm, making mothers feel more connected to their bodies and to the whole experience of pregnancy.

We also found that mindfulness can support mums-to-be in enhancing their relationship not just with themselves, but also with their partner and with their baby. Interestingly, we saw a significant increase in *both* expectant parents' wellbeing. Women demonstrated a significant improvement in symptoms of stress, anxiety, depression, pregnancy-related distress and labour worry; while their partners showed significant progress in managing anxiety and depression, as well as improvement in self-reported symptoms of perceived stress. Other studies that have underlined the positive, stress-reducing effect of mindfulness in pregnancy have proven that being relaxed in pregnancy is not only good for the mum-to-be but also for the baby (Newman *et al*, 2017; Sbrilli *et al*, 2020). Studies have even shown that mindfulness can help to take the sting out of a bad night's sleep (Felder *et al*, 2017).

So, as you can see, mindfulness has a lot going for it!

Getting the Most From This Book

This book is set out in five main chapters:

1. First Trimester (Weeks 0–12) – A Time to Adjust to the Idea of Pregnancy
2. Second Trimester (Weeks 13–28) – A Time to Enjoy and be Proud of Your Pregnancy
3. Third Trimester (Weeks 29–40) – A Time to Slow Down and Nurture Yourself
4. Labour and Birth – A Time of Transition
5. Parenthood – A New Way of Being

Each of these chapters will ...

- explore the main physical and emotional changes that you will be going through during this stage of the pregnancy journey, complete with "Key Mindful Intentions" for both you and your partner (whether the father of your baby, your life partner or another partner supporting you through your pregnancy; see page 11 for more on this)

- provide insight into how mindfulness can support you during this stage of your pregnancy and what techniques you might use to achieve this – whether focusing on the breath, the senses, everyday actions or other elements
- offer six mindfulness-focused practices for you to choose from
- end with a series of journaling starter questions – as inspiration for you to keep a mindful record of your pregnancy journey as you move through it, if desired

Although the six practices outlined within each of the five chapters are congruent with a particular stage of pregnancy (which means you can choose to work through them in the order suggested as you progress through your pregnancy), you may alternatively wish to dip in and out of the different chapters of the book to explore the mindfulness practices that simply feel right for you at any given time. It is entirely up to you.

Either way, each of the practices in the book has been designed to be as straightforward as possible and to fit into even the busiest of lifestyles. Mindfulness is simple, if not always easy.

Making the Time for Mindfulness

To begin with, I suggest that you simply set aside a few dedicated moments in your day to *intentionally* practise mindfulness – five minutes would be good if possible. Pick one of the 30 mindfulness practices that instinctively feels right for you – whether based on the chapter of the book that it's in, a title that appeals to you, the type of focus it requires (such as the breath, the senses or a visualization), or any other factor that draws you in. And simply follow the guidance on the page.

Once you become more familiar with the practices as you try them, you'll start to develop your own preferences, and your own natural flow in terms of what you choose to do when. You may then like to try extending your intentional practice to ten or ideally 20 minutes each day. If this feels like an unrealistic target for you, just do what you can and you will still benefit.

Being Kind to Yourself

It's important to treat yourself with kindness as you start your mindfulness practice; cultivating a practice is all about curiosity, patience, trust and self-compassion. As you progress, you will be able to use your mindfulness skills at any moment throughout your day as a way of reconnecting with the present moment, your body and your baby.

Involving Your Partner in Your Journey

Throughout the book we have taken into account the impact of pregnancy not only on you, as the mum-to-be, but also on partners and their role in supporting you. A partner may be the father of your baby, your life partner or a chosen pregnancy and birth companion, such as your mum, sister, a trusted friend or a doula – and you may have more than one. Whoever they are, connecting with them and sharing this book and the mindfulness practices in it, will help to support and sustain both (or all) of you as you move through pregnancy and birth – into parenthood.

Embracing the Power of Mindful Journaling

Expressive writing and journaling have been shown to have many benefits – both physical and psychological – such as improved mood, greater wellbeing, lower stress levels and fewer depressive symptoms, all of which are particularly beneficial during pregnancy and parenthood. It can therefore be helpful to make mindful journaling an integral part of your pregnancy journey.

Whether you're going through a good time, a tough time, or even an average time, taking a few moments now and again to reflect on your thoughts and feelings and note them down in a "journal" can help you to become more self-aware and to untangle thoughts and feelings from facts, which, in turn, can promote a sense of ease. Understanding that our thoughts and feelings are not permanent but are passing events that shift and change, just as life does, is an important element of bringing more mindfulness into our daily lives.

You can use a special journal for your musings if you want, but you don't have to have a special book – the important thing is to record your experiences and reflections in whatever form feels best for you. This can be done as and when you feel able, remembering that our connection with an event or feeling can soon fade, so more regular journaling will allow you to keep a clearer record.

To this effect, you will find some starter questions at the end of each of the five main chapters in the book which can be used, if desired, as prompts for your journaling during each stage of your journey to becoming a parent. Feel free to express yourself in any way as you do this – whether writing in full sentences, making lists, noting key words, drawing, colouring or anything else that represents how you feel in the moment.

Taken together, the collection of observations, insights, drawings and anything else that you include will create a rich record of your pregnancy, which can be rewarding to look back on once your pregnancy is over – a chance to reflect on your experience and take a moment to congratulate yourself.

So Let's Get Started

My hope is that this book will encourage you to take the time to slow down, be present and use the insight and practices that it offers as a mindful gift to yourself as you embark on this incredible journey toward motherhood.

I wish you all the very best for your pregnancy and beyond.

CHAPTER 1
FIRST TRIMESTER
(Weeks 0–12)

A TIME TO ADJUST TO THE IDEA OF PREGNANCY

Becoming pregnant is an "everyday miracle". You may wish to shout your news from the rooftops, you may find the first few weeks to be a time of reflection, or you may experience the news quite differently to how you imagined you would. The reality of pregnancy impacts everyone individually and uniquely. The one thing that's constant – whether your pregnancy is longed for or unexpected – is that it will bring about enormous change that will require you to make adjustments in your life.

In the first trimester, there are few obvious external signs of change. Despite this, it's a time when there are marked hormonal shifts. These shifts can bring a "pregnancy tiredness" that may feel all-consuming.

As your body adjusts to being pregnant, you may also experience nausea, sore breasts and/or unsettling cramps. In addition, the hormonal shifts play a part in making you feel far more emotional than may be usual for you.

However, the effect on your emotions is not just down to hormones. Your emotions will also be affected by your own personal history, emotional wellbeing and pregnancy history, which means that some psychological adjustment will be required. After all, your mental image of yourself – indeed your very identity – will start to change as the anticipation of your evolving pregnancy and pending motherhood begins, which is why it's so useful to have a technique like mindfulness at your disposal to help you keep a calmer, more even mind.

The impact of becoming pregnant will also ripple out and have an effect on how you view your relationships, career, financial situation and so on. Unsurprisingly, many women may feel a sense of loss and worry around this time, as well as excitement and anticipation about a new beginning. What can make it extra challenging is that all this happens at a time when you may want to keep news of your pregnancy quiet, which means that you may not have access to your normal support networks.

Key Mindful Intentions – For You, the Mum-to-be:

- Try to rest when you can and avoid booking in too many activities. It's OK to slow things down and take more breaks than you normally might.
- Try not to be too hard on yourself, no matter how things are unfolding. Not everyone enjoys how pregnancy affects their body and makes them feel.
- Take time to consider who is best placed to support you emotionally during your pregnancy journey. It isn't always

the most obvious person, so it might be a friend, family member or even a colleague. Be sure to connect with them regularly from the start and talk about how you are feeling – both the joys and the challenges.

- Take time to care for yourself from the get-go. Regularly doing things that you enjoy, that relax you and/or that provide you with gentle exercise will set you up well for the rest of the pregnancy journey ahead.
- Take time to talk with your partner about what you are both experiencing, as the excitement and anxiety of new pregnancy can bring about lots of changes in both your physical and emotional relationship.

Key Mindful Intentions – For Partners:

Invite and encourage your partner / birth partner to ...

- Take some time for themselves to process how they feel about the new pregnancy. Although they won't experience the same *physical* changes as you, there will be lots of *emotional* change for them, too.
- Think about what becoming a parent really means for them and how this is likely to affect their approach to things like work-life balance.

- Talk about what's going through their mind with their loved ones, including you.
- Take time to be with you and discuss how you can support each other over the coming weeks and months.
- Decide, together, when to share the news of the new baby with others.

How Can Mindfulness Help During This Stage of Pregnancy?

Regular mindfulness practice can help us to become less reactive, feel less stressed and have a more balanced perspective on life's challenges. It has been shown to decrease the production of the stress hormones cortisol and adrenaline, and promote the release of the feel-good hormone oxytocin, which means that by incorporating the techniques in this book into your everyday life during the first trimester of your pregnancy, you will be establishing a calmer environment for your baby to grow in – letting him or her know that they are safe and protected.

A 2018 study of expectant parents' use of mindfulness during pregnancy demonstrated that the majority experienced mindfulness as a valuable preparation for the challenges they met when they went through the life-changing events of becoming parents (Lönnberg *et al,* 2018). Practising, integrating and embodying mindfulness seems to foster the development of wisdom that allows you to better cope with the many challenges involved in pregnancy and impending parenthood.

As human beings, our minds often get drawn into "autopilot" thinking, where we can spend large amounts of our time not being truly aware of our present-moment experience. We're sure you have experienced setting out on a walk (or even a drive) somewhere only to arrive at your destination without any real memory of the journey or route you took, or have gotten so caught up in thinking about something that you forget to do something else important. When in such autopilot thinking, we are much more likely to react to situations based on past or future thinking, rather than respond to our actual present-moment experience.

While reflection on the past can be interesting and future planning can be helpful, without the awareness and ability to reconnect to the present through practices such as mindfulness, reflection can all too easily tip into unhelpful rumination at times, and future planning into over-thinking and anxiety – none of which are healthy at the best of times, never mind at the start of a new pregnancy.

Gently bringing your attention to the breath – as you breathe in and out – is a simple and valuable way to shift from autopilot thinking at any time. Doing this allows you to pause and gather a scattered mind, stabilize your attention and reconnect with the reality of your current experience, as a newly pregnant mum-to-be.

Quiet focus on the act of breathing has been used for centuries as a way to centre ourselves and has also been used for generations by midwives as a way to encourage calm during pregnancy and labour. As breathing is like a metronome that never stops, it is something that we can use as an anchor to the present moment.

The effect on both our minds and bodies as we slow down and intentionally focus awareness on the breath is profound: it allows us to step back from the usual chatter of our busy minds, it slows down our pulse rate and it makes space for us to settle and really notice what is going on in the present moment – in this case, within these first precious weeks and months of pregnancy.

A 2016 study on mindfulness and breathing found that even after just two weeks of attention-to-breath meditation training, participants were more effective in regulating aversive emotions associated with the stress response. (Doll *et al*, 2016).

It might seem very simple but the beauty of the breath is that it's always there for you. So any time that any aspect of your pregnancy might feel a little overwhelming and you need to take a "moment", you can simply take a few breaths in order to bring your attention to the here and now, when all you need to be is whatever, and wherever, you already are.

Self-compassion practices such as the "Well-Wishing Mantra" (see practice 5, page 37) can also be particularly helpful to ease any sense of overwhelm during this first stage of pregnancy, as the cultivation of an attitude of greater friendliness and openness can be uplifting and deepen a sense of good will and connection with both ourselves and others (Gentile *et al,* 2019).

Six Mindfulness Practices for the First Trimester

The practices that follow are an ideal introduction to mindfulness if you are new to it, and will reconnect you with some of the basics if you are already familiar with it. As well as offering practices that cultivate present-moment awareness of where you are on your pregnancy journey right now through placing attention on the *breath*, you will find practices that focus on the body's senses and also on the life-affirming practices of self-compassion and gratitude.

1

Mindful Breathing: It All Starts Here

If you've never tried mindfulness before, the easiest way to start is by intentionally focusing on your breath. It's a bit like squeezing the brakes on a bike – it slows you right down, allowing you to simply "be" in the moment, taking in the full remarkable experience of your current stage of pregnancy.

Sit comfortably somewhere nice and quiet, and allow yourself to arrive in this moment right here and now. That's it – you've started.

Bring your attention to the breath ...

As you breathe in, bring your attention fully to the
in-breath,
As you breathe out, bring your attention fully to the
out-breath,
Noticing the pauses in between the breaths.

Allow the breath to be as it is.
There's no need to change, direct or force it in any way.
Just allow the breath to flow.

Notice the sensation as the breath enters the body,
then leaves it again,
Notice it in the abdomen, the chest, the nostrils,
Focusing, perhaps, on where the sensation is most
vivid for you.

When you notice that your attention has wandered
away from the breath,
Be curious about what is pulling for your attention,
perhaps noticing any patterns that emerge.
Then, gently and kindly escort your attention back to
the breath,
Allowing it to anchor you in this present moment.

After a few minutes expand your awareness to
take in the whole of your body and breath,
And after a few moments expand your awareness
once more to take in the space around your body.
Sense your whole body resting and breathing in
this broad expanded awareness,
Noticing the sense of spaciousness that this
may bring.
As best you can, try to take a sense of this calm
spaciousness with you into the rest of your day.

If for any reason, or at any point in your practice, you
find the breath difficult to engage with, try shifting
the focus of your attention to your feet on the floor
and notice the sense of stability and steadiness that
arises from this connection.

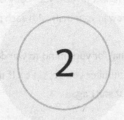

Counting Breaths: One to Nine

Intentionally being present for just nine consecutive breaths – one breath for each month of the pregnancy to come – can help to create a sense of increased space and calm if ever things feel like they're getting on top of you. This practice is particularly great if you don't have much time.

Simply place your attention fully on your breath as you breathe in and out nine times.

You can keep track on your fingers if it helps, whether counting out loud or inside your own head.

As you breathe, reflect on how your baby is going to be nurtured and grow in your belly with each passing month.

It's totally normal for your mind to wander or to lose track of which number you are up to. If that happens, don't worry; just start again.

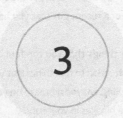

Tuning Into the Senses: Five Alive

This practice, designed for all of the senses to be used in one sitting, is a wonderful way to connect you to the present moment and an opportunity for you to give your baby information about the world. Placing awareness on the physical sensations of sight, touch, sound, smell and taste can be wonderfully grounding and stabilizing during this trimester full of lots of newness and adjustment.

- Notice five things that you can see.
  Bring your attention to five things around you that give a sense of the visual beauty of the world and that you would like your baby to see when it

33

arrives. Perhaps the blueness of the sky, the petals of a flower, or a recent gift that you have been given.

● Notice four things that you can feel.
Bring your attention to four things that you are currently feeling. Maybe a breeze on your face or the softness of a blanket in your hands.

● Notice three things that you can hear.
Bring your attention to three sounds that you can hear in the background. Perhaps the sound of rain, birdsong or a favourite piece of music.

● Notice two things that you can smell.
Bring your awareness to two scents in your vicinity. Maybe a bunch of fresh flowers, a pot of coffee, or, if you're outside, the smell of cut grass.

● Notice one thing that you can taste.
Bring your awareness to something that you can taste right now, in this moment. Perhaps by taking a sip of a drink, eating something, or just noticing the current taste in your mouth.

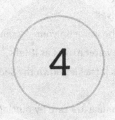

Connecting with the Senses: Sensational Shower

Something as simple as paying attention to the sensations we experience when showering is a great way to activate our parasympathetic nervous system, which is the part of our nervous system that enables us to rest and regenerate.

This is a particularly important system in your body to know how to access during this first trimester of pregnancy – in order to help maintain balance as you adjust to all the newness of your baby growing inside of you.

As you shower, take a moment to notice the various
sensations involved –
The feeling of the water on your skin and hair,
The sounds the water makes as it falls,
The look of it as it trickles down the shower screen ...

Give yourself some extra care by putting your hand on
any area of discomfort in your body and caressing it
gently –
In the same way that you will soothe your baby once it
is born as a loving parent.

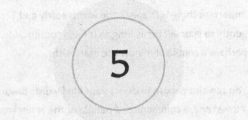

Practising Self-Compassion: Well-Wishing Mantra

Repeating specific positive words or phrases to yourself (sometimes called mantras) is a simple and effective way to practise mindfulness as well as to help build your capacity for self-compassion and kindness.

Sit comfortably, with one hand on your heart and one on your bump, and repeat these words out loud:

May you be happy and healthy,
May you be safe and protected,
May you live in peace and with kindness.

You can use wording of your own if you prefer. The important thing is to speak the words softly and gently to yourself for as long as it feels comfortable – perhaps a couple of minutes to start with.

You can also choose to direct your kind words toward a loved one, a community of people or the wider world if you want – as well as to yourself. See page 145 for a Well-Wishing Mantra specifically for your new baby.

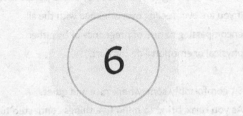

6

Counting Your Blessings: Gratitude is Good

Science tells us that a regular gratitude practice can have a profound effect on our brains, improving our sense of wellbeing by increasing the release of feel-good hormones dopamine and oxytocin.

This can be particularly helpful during the first trimester of pregnancy to help set you up well for the rest of the journey ahead – as it actively encourages you to acknowledge simple positive things that you might otherwise overlook, such as the day-to-day kindness of a hug.

This will help to give you a more balanced perspective if you are ever feeling overwhelmed with the all-encompassing nature of pregnancy or by either physical or emotional discomfort.

Sit comfortably somewhere nice and quiet.
As you relax, bring to mind five things connected to your baby or your experience of pregnancy that you are grateful for.

Feel free to take your time with this – to find what really resonates for you.

Count each one off on your fingers as you think of it.

Once you have all five, quietly reflect on them,
Letting yourself sit with the sensation of feeling grateful and noticing how it feels.

It's OK if you can't think of five things that you feel grateful for in the moment, if you can't think of *any*, or if feelings such as sadness, come up.

You're not doing anything wrong.

Simply bring your attention back to the physical
sensation of your breath and know that this is enough
– and you are enough, just as you are.

Starter Questions for Journaling in the First Trimester

If you like the idea explored in the Introduction of developing a regular mindful journaling practice to help you lean into the experience of each stage of pregnancy and keep a record of it, here are some questions to help you get started:

- How did you feel when you found out that you were pregnant? Was it how you expected to feel?

- In what ways can you feel your body start to change already? How does that make you feel?

- What is your greatest fear about this pregnancy? What things can you do to help overcome that fear?

- What feels good or gives you the greatest sense of joy about your pregnancy?

- What do you feel you need help with at the moment? And who might be best placed to give you this help?

Feel free to write or draw your answers in any form that naturally emerges; there is no right or wrong here.

Also feel free to ask your own questions and explore your own topics if you want – whether instead of or as well as these ones.

CHAPTER 2
SECOND TRIMES-
TER
(Weeks 13–28)

A TIME TO ENJOY AND BE PROUD OF YOUR PREGNANCY

In this second trimester of your pregnancy – months 4, 5 and 6 – your impending parenthood is likely to start to feeling more "real" as your bump begins to grow and show. For some, this time may also bring a sense of increased wellbeing as your energy levels recover from the fatigue, sickness and perhaps worry of the first few months. This is an ideal time to ensure that nourishing activities are part of your everyday life; establishing a healthy routine of self-care now will make it easier for you to maintain a habit of caring for yourself once you have a new baby to look after, too.

Perhaps one of the biggest changes during this stage of pregnancy is that you will begin to notice your baby moving. This may initially just be a small flutter, like butterflies in your tummy, but as your baby grows and becomes stronger, so too will the feelings of movement. This change offers the opportunity of connecting emotionally as well as physically with your baby. Beginning to build a strong sense of interconnectedness with your baby at this time is one of the first steps in the important process of bonding, and also provides a wonderful opportunity to get your partner involved in creating the foundations on which your new family identity will grow.

By the end of the second trimester, your baby will be listening to your voice, and will recognize it after birth.

You are likely to have been offered an ultrasound scan by the start of this trimester (at around 10–12 weeks) and also to be offered another one at around 20 weeks – when the sex of the baby can be determined if you wish to know. You may find that your own anticipation, coupled with curiosity from family and friends, creates pressure to find out and/or reveal whether you are having a boy or girl. Notice how you feel about this and how we can so easily be drawn into future-thinking and planning. Consider if knowing and/or sharing your baby's sex feels right for you and your partner, or if remaining in the present may be more helpful for you at this time. There is no right or wrong answer.

Seeing your baby on an ultrasound scan, hearing their heartbeat for the first time and feeling them move can be tremendously moving for both you and your partner, but can also bring up anxiety for some, as the reality of parenthood becomes even more real. Please know that this is not unusual, so if it's part of your experience, you are not alone. You might even be able to use the sense of responsibility that often comes with such feelings to positive effect, by channeling it into reflection on any positive lifestyle changes you might like to make for the sake of your baby.

The second trimester is also a good time to start preparing for the arrival of your baby. You could, for example, find out about what childbirth classes are running locally, explore your options for where to give birth, and consider how you want to feed your baby. As you start to plan, you may find yourself feeling more confident and in control.

Key Mindful Intentions – For You, the Mum-to-be:

- Keep things as slow as possible. This is a unique time, so, as best you can, try to take time out to relax, enjoy and savour it.
- Learn all you can about what to expect throughout the rest of your pregnancy and the birth, asking lots of questions so that you can make informed choices about the care you receive.
- Focus on making healthy lifestyle choices – as a sign of trust and respect for your body.
- Take time to share with your partner how you experience your baby growing and making themselves known to you inside your belly.
- Consider with your partner whether you want to know the sex of your baby and, if so, who you want share the news with.

Key Mindful Intentions – For Partners:

Invite and encourage your partner / birthing partner to ...

- Spend lots of time with you and be open and honest about how they are feeling – whether it's joy, fear or any other emotion.

- Accompany you to antenatal clinic visits and/or classes, and ask questions there. This will not only help you to feel more supported but will also help them to feel more informed and involved.
- Consider making some positive lifestyle changes, such as giving up smoking, cutting back on alcohol or coffee, or making generally healthier food choices.
- Reach out to other partners to share feelings and ideas. They might be able to meet other partners through childbirth classes, for example.
- Try to take some time for themselves – whether to exercise, visit friends, indulge in a hobby or whatever else nourishes them.

How Can Mindfulness Help During This Stage of Pregnancy?

Regular practice of mindfulness can really enrich the experience of pregnancy by allowing us to become more aware of all the changes taking place within us.

While our minds tend to get drawn into the past or future, our body – and its senses of sight, touch, sound, smell and taste – are always here, in the present moment. As our senses provide us with an ever-ready way of fully engaging with our present-moment physical experience, it makes them an invaluable tool for mindfulness practice.

As you learn to be more mindful of your sensations, your attention will be gently drawn away from thoughts and thinking, allowing you to connect with and appreciate all kinds of small things that you might otherwise overlook – whether that's how it feels to see your bump showing, how it feels when you touch your growing bump, or whether your sense of smell and taste is affected by your pregnancy, and so on.

Our body's senses also affect our emotions. For example, by tuning into our sense of touch, we can activate our parasympathetic nervous system, which produces the hormone oxytocin that encourages us to feel calm and relaxed. This is in contrast to the sympathetic nervous system, which is responsible for what is often known as our "fight or flight response" to fears and threats in life and, as such, releases adrenaline that causes our heart rate to rise, our breathing to become more shallow and us to feel stressed.

In a 2015 paper on the benefits of self-soothing, Swedish researchers describe how oxytocin is released in response to the activation of sensory nerves during labour, breastfeeding and sexual activity. They also describe how oxytocin is released in response to low-intensity stimulation of the skin, such as in response to touch, stroking, warm temperatures and other such sensations. Consequently, oxytocin is not only released during physical interaction between mothers and infants, but also during positive physical interaction between adults, and during positive physical interaction with ourselves, even if it's something as simple as running a finger over our lips or placing our hands on our pregnant belly. (Uvnäs-Moberg *et al*, 2015).

Once you become more aware of your body and your senses through mindfulness practices such as the ones that follow, you will gradually be able to embrace this sense of increased awareness in your daily life, too – both during pregnancy and beyond.

Six Mindfulness Practices for the Second Trimester

In mindfulness practice, connecting with the body and noticing sensations with an attitude of curiosity, non-judgement and just "allowing" are used as a way to build our capacity for moment-by-moment awareness. The main thread flowing through the practices that follow is on how tuning into, sensing and reconnecting with our bodies can benefit both our bodies and our minds, as well as deepen our connection with our growing baby.

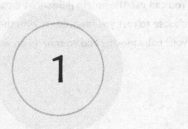

1

Connecting with Your Baby:
Hand on Belly, Hand on Heart

When you notice your baby move, place your left hand
on your belly and your right hand on your heart. Now,
focus your attention on your baby and take a moment
to simply "be" with both your breath *and* your baby.

This is a wonderful way for you to build a sense of
connection between yourself and your baby before he
or she is born.

It doesn't matter where you are or what you're doing;
when you feel movement, you can use it as a cue to
take a moment to connect and be mindful.

You can use the breath guidance on page 27 or simply choose to rest your awareness with the sensation of your baby moving and your hand on your heart.

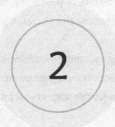

Caring for Yourself: Lotion Love

The next time you get out of the bath or shower, treat yourself to an application of some of your favourite body lotion or cream.

Pay particular attention as you apply the lotion or cream to your bump.

Take time to really notice all the sensations – of opening the cream, squeezing it into your hands, rubbing it into your bump, and how your skin feels as the cream is absorbed.

Notice, too, the texture of your bump, the tone of the skin there and anything else that stands out.

As well as making a soothing mindfulness practice, regular acts of self-care like this are a great way to help you to slow down, relax and enjoy this stage of your pregnancy more.

3

Observing Yourself: Body Scan

A body scan is a mindfulness technique that involves simply bringing your awareness to the different parts of your body, and any sensations occurring there, in a gradual sequence from one end of your body to the other.

It is common for people to feel tired or fall asleep during a body scan. So much so that some people even use the technique as a way of getting back to sleep if they waken at night. No matter what happens, try approaching the experience with a sense of compassion toward yourself; there is no right or wrong way to do it.

Although traditionally done lying down, this practice can also be done sitting or standing depending on what brings the most sense of comfort. It's OK for partners to lie flat on their backs if comfy but mums-to-be are best to lie on their left side, with perhaps a pillow between their legs and under their belly.

Sit, stand or lie comfortably with pillows to support your bump.

Close your eyes and bring your awareness to your body as a whole, feeling its weight and the points of contact it has with the ground.

Take a few deep breaths, noticing the sensations of breathing in your nose, throat, chest and abdomen.

Now slowly bring your attention down to your toes, noticing all the sensations that might be occurring there – cold, warmth, tingling, heaviness, or no sensation at all.

When you are ready, slowly move your attention gradually up your body – to your feet, ankles, calves, knees, thighs.

As best you can, gently notice the sensations you are experiencing in each area without judgement.

Slowly continue to work your way up the rest of your body – to your pelvis, lower back, belly, chest, upper back, shoulders, arms, neck, head and face, being curious about the sensations in each area as you journey through them.

See if it is possible to softly breathe into any area of discomfort, allowing a sense of softening and ease as you breathe out.

If you notice your mind wandering off, just gently gather your attention and return to noticing the sensations in your body.

Finally, imagine sending your breath all the way down to your feet and then back up again, as if your whole body were breathing.

Then, when you are ready, slowly open your eyes if they have been closed and gently begin to move your body.

Yoga Mamma: Child's Pose

Regular yoga benefits mums-to-be in all kinds of ways. It not only prepares the body for the physical demands of birth by promoting muscle strength and tone, but the nature of the practice can also provide a welcome chance to relax, helping to reduce stress and encouraging an active connection with the body. If your doctor hasn't advised you otherwise, consider trying a local pregnancy yoga class.

A pose that you can try yourself *at home* any time that you would like to relax and reconnect with your body is the classic wide-knee Child's Pose, which is also a wonderfully soothing way to take pressure off your back.

Kneel with the tops of your feet touching the floor and your bottom gently resting on your heels.
Place your knees wider than hip-width apart to allow space for your bump.
Gently bring your chest down toward the floor, letting your belly come between your legs.
Extend your arms in front of you, with your forehead resting on the floor.

You can support your forehead or chest with a folded blanket for comfort, particularly as your pregnancy progresses.

If this posture is not accessible for you, you can adapt it to fit your needs, such as by kneeling more upright and resting forward onto a chair.

As you hold the pose, be present and notice the sensations in your body.

It's fine if your mind wanders off; simply bring your attention back to the present moment, non-judgmentally and with kindness.

Then, when you're ready, gently come back up to sitting.

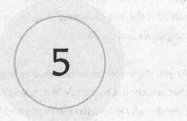

Getting Creative:
Make Something of Meaning

It can be lovely to engage your senses in the act of making something either for yourself or your baby while you are pregnant. And this can be a fun and fulfilling activity to do with your partner, too.

You might, for example, like to create a visual representation of the feelings or emotions you have for your developing baby or of what becoming a parent means to you.

Whatever you choose to create – a drawing, painting, collage or anything else – you can get inspiration either from online resources such as Pinterest, or you can do it the "old-fashioned" way, looking at images in magazines and the like.

As you make your artwork, contemplate each aspect that you choose to include in it, taking a moment to consider why it resonates with you and how it makes you feel.

If you feel like it, you can share your finished creation with friends or family and use it to start a conversation.

Alternatively, you might prefer to do something creative specifically for your baby. For example, you could write a special poem, make a belly cast, assemble their cot, decorate a picture frame or start to decorate their new room.

Whatever you choose to do, as you work, picture yourself being together with your baby, enjoying whatever it is that you are doing or making for them.

This process of painting a mental picture will help to build the sense of connection between you.

If you are working on a longer project, like decorating your baby's room, it can be helpful to try focusing on doing it mindfully for set periods, perhaps even just five minutes at a time.

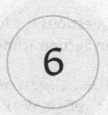

Enhancing Awareness: Mummy's Tummy

Actively observing and documenting your growing bump is an excellent way both to enhance a sense of general mindfulness during your pregnancy and to help you build a strong bond with your baby.

You can take photos, draw sketches, or even just regularly observe your bump.

The key is simply to spend a moment or two reflecting on your changing body and the baby growing inside you as regularly as you can – it truly is miraculous.

Starter Questions for Journaling in the Second Trimester

If you like the idea explored in the Introduction of developing a regular mindful journaling practice to help you lean into the experience of each stage of pregnancy and keep a record of it, here are some questions to help you get started:

- How did you feel when you first saw your baby on the ultrasound scan and/or when you first heard your baby's heartbeat? Who else was there? And how did it make you feel?

- Where were you when you first felt your baby move inside you? Who else was there? And how did it make you feel?

- **What is the first baby item that you have bought? Why did you choose this? How did it make you feel?**

- **Have you told anyone else about the pregnancy? If so, how did they react? How did their reaction make you feel?**

- **How would you describe the physical changes that you see in your body? How do these changes make you feel?**

Feel free to write or draw your answers in any form that naturally emerges; there is no right or wrong here.

Also feel free to ask your own questions and explore your own topics if you want – whether instead of or as well as these ones.

CHAPTER 3
THIRD TRIMESTER
(Weeks 29–40)

A TIME TO SLOW DOWN AND NURTURE YOURSELF

Through the last months and weeks of your pregnancy, your baby, and of course your bump, will steadily grow larger and larger. During these weeks, your body is therefore likely to start naturally slowing down; tiredness may return, and ordinary things like exercise, sleeping comfortably or activities in the home might become awkward.

As such, the third trimester is a time when you may well need more support from those around you – both physically and emotionally. It's a time to ask for – and accept – help when you need it. In short, it's a time to be as kind to yourself as possible.

Practising kindness toward ourselves can feel uncomfortable if we're not used to it, but research suggests that opening up to kindness has very significant effects on the degree of wellbeing that we experience, as well as on levels of creativity and of resilience when working through life's challenges.

So during this trimester in particular, try to be kind to your body by resting, napping and sleeping as much as you need to. Try to do something every day – no matter how small – that gives you a feeling of happiness, calm and/or joy. Take time every day to connect with and visualize your baby. Embrace your "nesting" instinct as much as you feel the need to. And also try your best to make time for your partner – time when you can just "be" together without trying to accomplish anything in particular.

Late pregnancy can be a challenging time as you may find that, as the final weeks of your pregnancy approach, worries about labour and birth become more prevalent. The birth stories of family, friends and people in the media can all add to a sense of uncertainty and fear.

Communicating openly and honestly with your partner and those closest to you about your fears, hopes and beliefs, can often help to bring more clarity and calm to the situation. Attending childbirth classes can also be useful as this allows you to learn from experts about the birth process, and writing down your preferences and intentions for the birth and the first few days after your baby is born is also likely to help you feel more prepared, empowered and confident.

Key Mindful Intentions – For You, the Mum-to-be:

- If you need more help with daily tasks during this stage, or a little more reassurance and support, be sure to ask for it. It is perfectly OK to ask for help and invite in more kindness when you need it.

- Take time to notice which activities deplete your energy or add to your worries, and which ones nourish you and provide a sense of calm and balance. Reduce the former; increase the latter.
- Be sure to keep building a network of compassionate support for yourself – connecting with your partner, family, friends and other expectant women and couples as desired.
- Discuss your hopes and preferences for labour and birth with your partner, noticing any attachment that either of you may hold to particular outcomes.
- Take time every day to bring loving, compassionate self-awareness to your body and your growing baby inside your belly – connecting to how you are in the moment, and building confidence and trust in yourself.

Key Mindful Intentions – For Partners:

Invite and encourage your partner / birthing partner to ...

- Ask what you need at any given time, but also try to anticipate and be proactive about emerging needs.
- Learn about labour and birth in general, and also about what you do and don't want during the process – so that they feel more confident about supporting you when the time comes.

- Join in with your maternal "nesting", whether by decorating the baby's room or doing anything else that you both feel drawn to do in preparation for your baby's arrival.
- Discuss the options in terms of how much time you can each take off work around the birth, and ensure that arrangements are in place for this.
- Talk openly – whether to you, family, friends or whoever else – reminding them that if the thought of being a parent still doesn't feel real or feels strange, to not be afraid to say so.

How Can Mindfulness Help During This Stage of Pregnancy?

Mindfulness can be an invaluable tool in the final trimester of pregnancy, particularly if you're feeling a lot more tired than before and/or preoccupied with worries about the birth. It can help to bring you out of your thinking and worrying mind, and back into the present moment, where you can observe and accept things as they are, rather than getting caught up in how you think they "should be" or "might be".

You may find that the late stages of pregnancy makes sitting still for any length of time uncomfortable. But the good news is that being mindful doesn't always have to involve sitting still.

You can bring your attention to the present moment in many ways, including by intentionally focusing on everyday tasks.

Turning ordinary activities, such a brushing your teeth, doing the dishes or making a cup of tea, into mindful activities is a great way of adding some mindful practice to a daily routine. It's also a useful way to introduce mindfulness to your life if you or your partner feel in any way uncomfortable, or perhaps unsure, about the more formal practices such as sitting and focusing on your breath or visualizations.

What matters is to be in the present moment; how you get there is less important. A 2015 study that used neuro-imaging techniques to show the effect that mindfulness practice has on the brain found that it enhanced attention, improved emotion regulation and also reduced stress. (Tang, 2015).

Cultivating present-moment awareness through the practice of mindfulness also helps us to choose where we place our attention, stopping us from getting so easily caught up in unhelpful thoughts and stories, which can be particularly useful if we are experiencing any anxiety during this final trimester in the lead-up to labour and birth. Learning to recognize and observe patterns of worry or self-judgement without giving them authority is a way to weaken their hold on us.

The use of speaking and listening as part of a mindfulness practice (see practice 6 on page 97) can also be especially helpful to deepen connection with partners and bring more awareness and understanding to the nature of our hopes, fears and beliefs at a time when we know that much in our lives is about to change. Being able to frame important conversations in a way that brings insight and awareness to whether the beliefs we hold are part of our core value system, or whether they represent learnt or adopted beliefs, can provide a more open, creative and ultimately more enjoyable life experience, as well as end stage of pregnancy.

Six Mindfulness Practices for the Third Trimester

Many of the practices that follow are about being kind, compassionate, caring and nurturing toward both you and your baby as you prepare for birth. They also aim to build mindful connections as you approach the day of your baby's arrival – your connection with yourself and the sensations you experience, with your baby who's now able to hear you in there, and also with your partner and/or birthing companion so that you both feel as comfortable as possible in the last months and weeks of the pregnancy.

A Quick Way to Relax: Go Slow

Do you sometimes find that being pregnant makes it a bit more difficult to do things as quickly as you did before? Great – if so, go with it! You can use it to your advantage, as a focus for mindfulness.

Whatever you are doing, deliberately slow it down and reflect on how it feels. It could be anything: eating, walking, tidying up, stroking a pet, even reading this book. As we slow down, we notice the present moment much more. Whatever feelings come up, just notice and – as best you can – accept them without judging. Then, gently bring your attention back to the present.

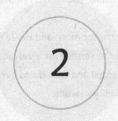

2

Magic in the Mundane:
A Daily Brush with Mindfulness

Turning a basic daily task into a mindful activity is
not only a great way for parents-to-be to add a little
more self-compassionate awareness to their day; it is
also enormously helpful training for the many routine
tasks involved in baby care.

Activities like nappy-changing, feeding, soothing and
bathing will all be repeated hundreds of times, so
will become wonderful opportunities for practising
mindfulness once your baby is born.

For now, try brushing your teeth mindfully.

Stay present in the moment and really focus your
attention on all the sensations involved:
The feel, taste, smell and sound and even how you
look as you do it if you want.

It sounds simple but notice how many times your
mind wanders off just in the few minutes that it takes
to brush your teeth.

And each time that this happens, it's a perfect
opportunity to train yourself to kindly bring your mind
back to the simple task in hand.

Connecting with Your Bump: Regular Playtime

Each time your baby gets active, you can use it as a cue for some momentary mindfulness.

Each time he or she gives a little kick, you could playfully give your belly a gentle rub or a little nudge and imagine that you're giving your baby a high five.

It's fun, and even a small smile or chuckle from you will trigger dopamine, endorphins and serotonin, making you feel happy and calm – which your baby will feel too.

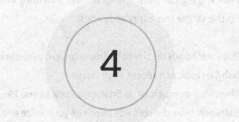

4

Sharing with Your Bump:
Your Baby's First Lullaby (or Story)

Your baby's hearing is developing all the time; from about 23 weeks they can hear your heartbeat. They will also start to hear sounds from the outside world, so hearing your voice during your pregnancy will really help your baby to feel attached to you when they are born.

This practice encourages you to mindfully talk or sing to your growing baby in your belly and can be an especially useful exercise for partners to do too, as it helps them to connect more with your baby and begin to build a bond of their own with them.

Plus, singing has been shown to have a calming effect on the singer too. Everybody wins!

Put your hands on the baby bump and visualize your baby, or look at a recent scan image.
Then sing as much, or as little, of a song as you like.
Baby will hear the soft vibrations of your voice and, if you sing the same song once they're born, they will recognize it and should find it comforting.

If singing is not for you, choose a story that you love.
Sit comfortably, then simply read it to your bump.
As you read, really try to imagine your baby, whether it's their squidgy thighs or the sensation of what it will feel like when they grab your finger.

If you can manage to read the story regularly, just as with singing, baby will become accustomed to your voice – the most significant sound they'll hear while in your womb. Research shows that babies' heart rates slow when you speak – they find it calming.

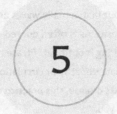

Exploring Sensations: Chill Out, Literally

This practice is adapted from the ice practice described by Nancy Bardacke in her book *Mindful Birthing*; it can be done individually or with your chosen birth companion. Just to be clear, we're not suggesting that holding ice is any way equivalent to labour pain but the idea of the practice is to encourage you to just "be with" discomfort, exploring what it truly feels like, rather than what we think it will feel like.

While the intense sensations might not change too much in themselves, with mindful attention, our relationship with them is likely to shift – just

like the contraction that might feel like it's going
to last forever but that actually waxes and wanes
in spells of intensity. As is often quoted: "Pain is
inevitable, suffering is optional." Please note: if you
have peripheral neuropathy or circulation problems,
such as Raynaud's disease, this practice may not be
appropriate for you.

Put some ice cubes in a bowl.
Take a moment to become still, bringing your attention
to the sensation of your breath as it flows in and out.

After a minute, take a handful of ice cubes and hold
them for 60–90 seconds, similar to the length of a
contraction in labour, noticing what happens both in
your mind and on your skin.

After 60 seconds, or if it becomes too uncomfortable
at any point, put the ice down and gently warm
your hands.
Return to focusing your attention on your breath for a
couple of minutes before once again picking up the

ice for another 60–90 seconds, mimicking the flow
of contractions through labour.

While you hold the ice, allow your attention to focus
on the flow of your breath, or you may wish to bring
a sense of curiosity and compassion to explore the
sensations you are experiencing:
The cold stinging, the hard edges, the slow trickle of
the ice as it melts ...
Pay attention to the story that your mind is telling
you about these sensations and notice any emotional
responses that you have.

When you feel ready, end the practice by disposing of
the ice and drying your hands on a warm towel.

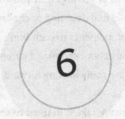

Time to Talk: Speak and Listen, Mindfully

This practice can provide an incredibly useful way of speaking and listening to anyone you love without judgement, criticism or interruption, while being fully aware of your own internal thoughts and reactions. It can be a particularly useful way of communicating with your partner or chosen birth companion as it creates a dedicated safe space to share openly with one another in the most mindful of ways.

In the following guidance, we have chosen to explore what the prospect of parenting means to you both. However, you could apply the same approach to

all kinds of issues or feelings that you and/or your partner normally find daunting or challenging.
Take a few quiet moments to each think of one thing that worries you about becoming a parent and one thing that you are really looking forward to.

When you are ready, take it in turns to share what you have thought of.

This means one person fully, mindfully listening while the other person is fully, mindfully speaking, and then swapping roles.

The key when listening is not to give in to any urge to respond, "jump in" or try to "fix" anything.

And the key when speaking is to drop all expectations of, or need for, a response or feedback.

Once you've done this, take a few quiet moments to each observe the thoughts, feelings and body sensations that came up for you when you were speaking and also when you were listening.

Each consider with attention how it felt to talk about something that you are worried about, as well as how it felt to share something positive.

Then, when you both feel ready, thank each other before continuing with the rest of the day.

Starter Questions for Journaling in the Third Trimester

If you like the idea explored in the Introduction of developing a regular mindful journaling practice to help you lean into the experience of each stage of pregnancy and keep a record of it, here are some questions to help you get started:

- Right now, how does the pregnancy feel, and how do you feel?

- What five reasons do you have to feel grateful for your partner, or anyone else particularly helping to support you through this time?

- How are you preparing your baby's space? What drew you to the things you have selected?

- If you had a baby shower, who came and what gifts did you receive?
- What are five ways in which you feel you are going to be a good parent?

Feel free to write or draw your answers in any form that naturally emerges; there is no right or wrong here.

Also feel free to ask your own questions and explore your own topics if you want – whether instead of or as well as these ones.

CHAPTER 4
LABOUR AND BIRTH

A TIME OF TRANSFORMATION

For most women, the third trimester ends – and labour usually starts – sometime between weeks 37 and 42. By this time your baby is considered fully grown and ready to be born.

Toward the end of your pregnancy, you may start to notice physical signs that your body and your baby are preparing for birth: you will still feel your baby move but they will come to a more settled position; you may sense that they have moved lower in your tummy; and you may become aware of "practice" contractions. All these new sensations can add to a sense of excitement and anticipation. It's not long now until you will meet your baby.

It's also very usual for the imminence of labour and birth to fuel feelings of uncertainty. Throughout our lives we face unknowns, and most of us like to be prepared for the future and feel that we have some control over what is happening to us. But it is unlikely that you will be able to control all aspects of labour and birth. For example, you may well not know when labour will begin. If you find that your feelings of joyful anticipation or happy planning start to shift toward overthinking, anxiety or even catastrophizing, try to step back and take a moment to simply notice that your feelings have changed. This simple act of noticing your changing feelings can be incredibly empowering. The awareness can provide you with a sense of choice about your feelings that you may not have thought you had.

Taking a little time to reflect on your birth intentions, noticing any sense of attachment or fixed expectation, and being open to the possibility of change can be extremely helpful. Birth is a fluid and transformative experience. It can be very straightforward and simple, but it can also be messy and complicated; it is always emotional and often not as we imagine. Remain positive in your hopes for birth, and allow kindness and compassion for yourself and your baby to guide your intentions. And remember that the experience of seeing your child being born will be as life-changing for your partner, if you have one, as it is for you, so be sure to share in the experience with them as much as possible.

Always try to be guided by your own knowledge and intuition, rather than fear. It can be helpful to use the mnemonic "BRAIN", with each letter of the word acting as a prompt for you or your birth companion to ask a question each time a big decision has to be made: Benefit, Risk, Alternatives, Intuition, Now?

For example, if your obstetrician is suggesting that your labour be induced, you may want to ask him or her:
B: "What is the Benefit to me and the baby?"
R: "What are the Risks of this?"
A: "What are the Alternatives?"
I: "Does this Intuitively feel right for me?"
N: "Does this have to be done Now?"

Key Mindful Intentions – For You, the Mum-to-be:

- Choose a positive mantra, or affirmation, that will help you to feel strong and powerful through labour and birth.
- Ensure that you know who you want to be surrounded by when you go into labour, whether your partner, a trusted friend or relative and/or a doula.
- Remain open as best you can to adjusting your intentions as your labour unfolds.
- Don't be afraid to ask questions of the people around you to help you feel reassured.
- Be sure to treat yourself with love and compassion throughout the process.

Key Mindful Intentions – For Partners:

Invite and encourage your partner / birthing partner to:

- Recognize how invaluable their role is in all this; although they are likely to be experiencing feelings of uncertainty, helplessness and fear, just as you might be, you will find strength in continuing to share with one another and support one another.
- Take responsibility for remembering items that you might need during labour, such as your phone charger or a music playlist.

- Look after themselves as well as you – so that they can be their best selves for you during labour. For example, pack a bag for themselves with some snacks, drinks and a change of clothes.
- Take the initiative, if required, in supporting your intentions and coping methods as labour unfolds, such as engaging with any breathing, relaxation or mindfulness practices that you have planned to use.
- Be mindful of things that they can say to support you, such as telling you how proud they are of you and reminding you how much they love you.

How Can Mindfulness Help During Labour and Birth?

The mind–body connection has a significant impact on how smoothly labour may flow. We are conditioned to automatically protect ourselves from pain; the unconscious response to the perceived "threat" of pain is resistance and fear. These feelings trigger our sympathetic nervous system to produce adrenaline, our "fight-or-flight" hormone, which has the direct effect of reducing the efficacy of contractions and slowing labour.

By learning the mindfulness skill of moment-by-moment awareness, you will find that you are better able to attune yourself with the rhythms of labour, trust the natural progressive stages, notice resistance as it arises and ground yourself in present-moment stability. From this steadiness, the body can engage the parasympathetic nervous system. This releases the feel-good hormone oxytocin, creating feelings of increased trust, self-compassion, self-efficacy and relaxation, therefore allowing labour to flow.

Mindfulness skills can also help us to develop the ability to really tune into and notice what our body is telling us and become more aware of how our mind is interpreting the body's messages. Pregnant women who practise mindfulness report that when they learn to relate differently to the negative thoughts that surround intense physical sensations, they cease to be so overwhelmed by feeling unable to cope with the pain, and are less fearful of losing control (Duncan *et al*, 2017).

Mindfulness also encourages us to practise noticing when our thoughts of wanting things to be a certain way lead to a sense of striving and expectation that are unlikely to be helpful in labour. It teaches us to be more open to how things are (rather than how we wish they were), inviting a sense of allowing, and encouraging kindness and self-compassion toward ourselves, especially at times when we may find ourselves feeling challenged or overwhelmed, such as during the birthing process.

Six Mindfulness Practices for Labour and Birth

The following practices build on what you have been learning and practising over the last few months. They are intended to give you active useful tools on which to draw as you go through the empowering, challenging and hugely transformative process that is labour and birth.

The Power of Self-Affirmation: Calming Mantra

A mantra, or affirmation, is a positive word or short phrase that you repeat over and over, as a powerful point of focus for your mind. Using a mantra during labour can help to bring increased calm and confidence. There are no rights or wrongs when creating one; simply use whatever works best for you. Here are some simple suggestions but feel free to come up with your own:

- (As you breathe in) *Calm,* (as you breathe out) *Open*
- *I trust myself, I can do this*
- *I am safe, my baby is safe*

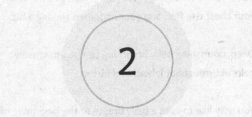

Blissful Breathing: It Starts in the Belly

The nourishing art of belly breathing involves taking deep breaths in through your nose down, through your chest and deep down into your belly (rather than higher up, in your chest), and then breathing out from deep in your belly up through the chest and out through your mouth.

You can practise knowing where your breath is coming from by placing your hand on your belly and feeling the rise and fall.

If you're breathing from your belly, you will feel your belly rise first or at the same time as your chest.

But if you're breathing from your chest, you will feel your chest rise first and your abdomen sinking a bit.

Deep, nourishing belly breathing can be immensely helpful throughout labour and birth.

You may like to take a belly breath at the beginning of each contraction and then again once the contraction is over.

It's worth bearing in mind that if you make your out-breath longer than your in-breath it will help to trigger your parasympathetic nervous system, which will allow oxytocin to flow and encourage relaxation.

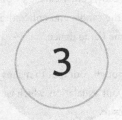

The Calm of the Out-Breath:
Dancing Candle

In the run-up to your due date, it can be helpful,
particularly in moments of worry or overwhelm,
to take a little time out for yourself. The simple
candlelight practice below is a useful one to
do during such moments.

Light a candle and place it on a table in front of you.

Watch the flame and take a couple of breaths in
and out to centre yourself.

Once you feel ready, gently exhale through your mouth toward the candle and notice the way your breath makes the flame dance.

Blowing out through your mouth makes it easier for you to extend your exhalation, which will help you to relax and stay calm.

Some mothers like to recall this image as their baby is being born – as a way to help them focus on the present moment and remain calm and in control.

4

Nurturing Visualization: Breath Hug for Your Baby

This beautiful breath visualization, which can easily be done anywhere, allows you to picture in your mind's eye your baby feeling loved, safe and warm – ready to come out and meet you when the time is right.

Place one hand on your belly and the other hand on your heart.

Take a moment to relax, closing your eyes if you want.

As you breathe, imagine your breath flowing around your baby as if you were wrapping them in a warm blanket.

Imagine your breath nourishing your baby as you breathe in and hugging your baby as you breathe out.

Empowering Visualization:
Thinking Helps Doing

Visualization techniques are a great way to reduce fear, release tension, promote relaxation and even reduce pain.

As your due date approaches, you may find it empowering to visualize the birthing process – to engage with how your amazing body is going to bring your baby into the world.

If this feels like it could be helpful for you, sit or lie somewhere comfortable, take a few deep breaths to centre yourself and imagine your cervix softening and opening, your body guiding your baby, and your baby moving down through the birth canal and coming out to meet you.

Another option is to visualize a peaceful location – one that makes you feel particularly calm, relaxed and ready to take on anything.
Spend as long as you like here, breathing in the sense of calm and peace.

The beauty of this practice is that it can be done anywhere, any time – even during labour if you find it helpful.

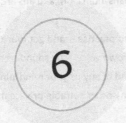

6

The Power of Sound: Let it Out

It's natural to vocalize during labour: it helps to empower you, relax your body and focus your energy.

It's not unusual to feel a little inhibited at first but it's not a matter of forcing yourself to make sounds; rather it's about giving yourself permission to do so.

Labour is a time to follow your instincts and let your body take over.

Low, deep sounds as you exhale on a long breath are best.

So moans, groans, hums, om and ahs are all good.

You may like to practise – and get more used to the sound of your own voice – by sounding a long deep "Om" at the end of any of your mindfulness practices, or indeed in any other suitable private moments.

Starter Questions for Journaling in the Run-Up to Labour

If you like the idea explored in the Introduction of developing a regular mindful journaling practice to help you lean into the experience of each stage of pregnancy and keep a record of it, here are some questions to help you get started:

- How are you feeling about the upcoming birth? If you have any concerns, what practical things can you do to help to overcome them?

- What are five ways that you would like to be supported during the birth?

- What have been some of the highlights of your pregnancy? Has it been different from what you expected?

- What does it feel like for your bump to be this big? What do you feel when you look in the mirror?

- Think of some of the ways that your partner, family or friends have helped or supported you throughout your pregnancy. How has that support made you feel?

Feel free to write or draw your answers in any form that naturally emerges; there is no right or wrong here.

Also feel free to ask your own questions and explore your own topics if you want – whether instead of or as well as these ones.

CHAPTER 5
PARENTHOOD

A NEW WAY
OF BEING

A NEW WAY
OF BEING

Over the last nine months your body and mind have gone through enormous change and, with the birth of your baby, this transition continues. Your body now needs time to recover; and, emotionally, you will need time to adjust to your new identity as a parent.

Bonding with your baby may feel immediate, instinctive and natural, or you may find that the process of getting to know your baby and the appreciation of this deep-embedded love grows more slowly. Both are fine, both are natural. This time is all about adjustment; life as you once knew it has changed, and adaption takes patience, trust and self-compassion.

Becoming a parent is a steep learning curve for most, and the reality of parenting can loom up on you suddenly when you bring your newborn home. But everyone's lives are different, so the ways in which you adjust and the time it takes to ease into this new way of being will be unique to you. As best you can, try not to judge yourself or compare yourself to others. Let your focus be on looking after yourself, your new baby and your family.

Throughout pregnancy you have worked hard to create a healthy, calm, connected and compassionate state of being in order to give your baby the best environment in which to grow. These intentions are equally as important as you navigate the first few weeks after the birth, and there is growing evidence that if you have practised mindfulness through pregnancy, it will have enduring benefits for your wellbeing post-birth (Sbrilli *et al,* 2020).

As a new parent, you are going to experience many moments of pure joy as well as many times when you feel utterly exhausted and overwhelmed. For most, the level of emotional fluctuation will be all-consuming during the first while and things will then gradually start to ease, but it's important to remember that if feelings of overwhelm, sadness, hopelessness, guilt, self-blame or depression persist, there are professionals available to support you. It's important to recognize that partners can suffer from postnatal depression, too, so if anyone is suffering, don't be worried or embarrassed about seeking the help needed for the wellbeing of you and your family.

This is a time for parents to hold your baby as much as possible – and to wonder and marvel. You can't do this too much; it's what babies need. When you hold your baby, they will feel loved and safe, so make the most of this time, as, before you know it, they will be off crawling, walking and running.

Key Mindful Intentions – For You, the Mum-to-be:

- Get as much rest as you can – whenever you can. Even if you can only sleep when the baby sleeps, and even if this is only a few short periods of rest several times a day, these minutes add up.

- Don't try to multitask. In the first few weeks, simply focus on taking care of your baby and taking care of yourself.

- Accept only the help that you need – and that you can see will truly be helpful. Although well intentioned, not all offers of help are needed or welcome during this time of all-encompassing newness.

- Every day, try to find at least a little time to connect with your partner, a friend and/or a family member about something other than your baby.

- Try your best to get outside, take a short walk or do at least ten minutes of stretching or yoga every day.

Key Mindful Intentions – For Partners:

Invite and encourage you partner / birthing partner to ...

- Arrange for the maximum time possible off work to be at home and help look after both you and the baby; you will need your partner now more than ever before.

- Manage visitors to the house: boundaries can be difficult to put in place when your loved ones are excited to meet your new arrival, but it's good to make sure the focus is firmly on you and your baby's need for rest during this period.

- Get involved as much as possible in the daily care of the baby. The more actively involved in your baby's everyday needs each carer is, the faster baby-care skills will develop and the faster confidence will grow.

- Talk with you about how your daily lives and relationship have changed – both for better and for worse – and discuss how you can support each other as your baby grows.

- Notice, enjoy and relish every new experience with your baby, considering what kind of parent and family member they want to be moving forward, what aspects of the way they were parented they might want to emulate and what they might do differently.

How Can Mindfulness Help Now That Your Baby Has Been Born?

Mindfulness is one of the best ways to manage the sometimes overwhelming complexity of post-birth emotions. You can use it as a way of connecting with your moment-by-moment experience and remaining present with your baby.

For example, try really tuning into your baby's needs when feeding. It may be tempting to use the time to "zone out", to watch TV or to check your phone, but feeding is a great time to practise mindful awareness. As you connect with your breath and focus on your baby, you will learn more quickly to notice and recognize their communication cues even though they cannot yet speak.

Another example of an everyday occurrence that can be used as a chance for mindfulness is when your baby cries – this can be the perfect opportunity to practise Mindful Walking to soothe both you and your baby (see practice 2 on page 139).

By reconnecting time and time again with a present-moment awareness, you will find, as in labour, that the intensity of difficulties is transient, that there are spaces of ease in between, and that there is much joy to be noticed and embraced.

Parenting requires constant interactions and decisions between you and your baby, and when we stay present, we make wiser choices. It is suggested that parents who can remain aware and accepting of their child's needs through using mindfulness practices can create a family context that allows for more enduring satisfaction and enjoyment in the parent–child relationship (Duncan *et al*, 2009). So let your baby, and any other children

you may have, be your mindfulness teachers! If we can pay
moment-by-moment attention to their cues and respond to them
with kindness, we will be shaping how they develop, as well as
teaching them to be able to do the same for themselves and others
in the future.

Mindfulness helps us to notice and accept all of our experiences. It
does not try to avoid the difficult or only highlight the wonderful; it
supports an open, compassionate curiosity to life that encourages
us to be more fully present in every moment. And this is what your
baby needs – your present, moment-by-moment love.

Six Mindfulness Practices for After Your Baby is Born

The mindfulness practices that follow are designed to nourish
and sustain you as you transition into parenthood. They not
only provide ways for you to bond with your baby but also offer
techniques that will empower you to remain as grounded as
possible throughout this time of immense change and wonder.

Baby-Gazing: Skin-to-Skin

Holding your new baby skin-to-skin as often as possible will help them to transition into the world, soothing and calming them as they get used to their new environment. And taking time to observe your baby and notice all the small changes that take place as each day passes will help you to be more fully present in their lives.

Dedicate a little time each day to holding your baby against your bare skin.
Feel the sensation of their skin on yours and observe all the tiny details about them:

Their hair, their smell, the folds of their skin, their tiny fingernails.
Take note of how these are gradually changing.

You might also want to intentionally talk to them as this will further encourage the connection between you.

Observe your own feelings as you do this practice.

The child is a wonder, and so are you.

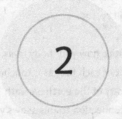

2

Mindful Walking: Step-by-Step

When we walk, we are often on autopilot. We tend to focus on our destination or things that we need to get done, with little awareness of what is going on either around us or in our bodies. However, if we use the experience of walking to provide a mindful connection to the present moment, it can allow us to slow down, find steadiness, embrace composure, and reconnect with a sense of inner calm and balance.

Mindful walking can be particularly useful when settling a crying baby. They will pick up on your heart rate, breathing and other such physical factors, so the

more calm and relaxed you are, the more calm and
relaxed they will be, too.

As you walk, notice how your body feels.
Feel the contact of each foot as it touches the ground.
Notice the solidity of the earth beneath your feet
and how your connection to this allows you to feel
grounded and stable.

Observe your body – and the flowing breath that
sustains it – as you move into each new step.
Pay attention to how your legs, feet and arms feel with
each forward movement.

With openness and curiosity, notice any sensations,
thoughts or feelings that arise, without lingering on
anything in particular.

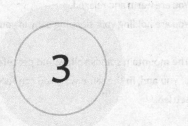

3

Strengthening and Stabilizing Visualization: Mindful Mountain

The practice of visualization, or focusing your attention on something in your mind's eye, can allow you to enhance all sorts of positive attitudes depending on what visual you choose to focus on, what this suggests to you and what it makes you feel. So if, for example, you were to focus on the image of a mountain, you might tap into feelings of stillness, strength, stability and/or beauty.

Bring your attention to your breath.

Imagine you are gazing at a beautiful, mighty mountain.

You are warm and relaxed.
You are holding your sleeping baby in your arms.

The mountain stands solidly and peacefully in front
of you and, in the same way, you can feel calm and
settled.

As you recognize the great strength and stability of
the mountain before you, know that you, too, have the
capacity to embody this type of centred, unwavering
stillness in the face of all that changes in life – over
the hours, the days and the years.

As you breathe, allow a deep feeling of relaxation and
love to envelop you and your baby.
It cocoons you both and makes you feel safe.

Just as the mountain will endure, so will your love:
Unchanging, unwavering, rock solid.

Forever.

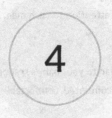

4

The Power of Touch: Baby Massage

Daily baby massage is a lovely interactive way to start a mindfulness practice with your baby.

Research has suggested that the possible benefits of baby massage include enhanced bonding, better sleep/relaxation, a positive boost in the hormones that control stress, and reduced crying.

Find a comfortable spot for both you and your baby. Start by very gently rubbing his or her head with the pads of your fingertips.

Then move slowly and gradually down their little body, paying mindful attention to each main area until you reach their feet.

Be sure to tune in to your baby's responses, noticing if they're calm, contented, comfortable, alert, fussy or whatever else.

The massage can last as long as both you and your baby are enjoying it.

5

Sharing the Love:
Well-Wishing Mantra for Your Baby

We all have a lot of internal dialogue going on inside our minds. But when we are feeling exhausted or emotionally vulnerable, which a lot of people often are during the first stages of new parenthood, this internal "chatter" can all too easily become negative and judgemental if we're not careful. Research has shown that the volume of our internal critic can be turned down through a mindfulness practice known as "well-wishing".

You may have already tried the "Well-Wishing Mantra" practice during the first trimester of your pregnancy (see page 37), and, if you enjoyed this, you may still find it useful to do now.

But you might also like to try one specifically for your baby now that he or she has arrived.

So, the next time you notice yourself feeling frustrated, overwhelmed, self-critical or any other less-than-positive thoughts or emotions, see if you can replace them with some more loving thoughts by repeating the following well-wishing mantra to your baby:

> *Welcome to family,*
> *Welcome to love,*
> *Welcome to happiness,*
> *Welcome to our lives.*

You can use wording of your own if you prefer. The important thing is to speak the words softly and gently for as long as it feels comfortable – perhaps a couple of minutes to start with.

Day-to-Day Mindfulness: Embrace the Moment

Once your baby is born it may seem impossible to find the time or space you feel you need to practise mindfulness. Fortunately, as we also explored during the third trimester, the good thing about mindfulness is that the intention to bring more present-moment awareness to your experience can be brought to any daily activity.

This means that even if you don't have much time spare, you can still practise by doing simple activities with a mindful approach. Almost anything can be done mindfully, whether taking a shower, making and drinking a cup of tea or coffee, feeding your baby or changing your baby.

All you need to do is slow down and intentionally focus your attention on the present moment.

Here are a few other tips that will help you to move through each day in as mindful a way as possible, paying conscious, compassionate attention to each moment as it unfolds:

- When you wake up in the morning, visualize the day ahead and set an intention for how you'd like it to go. This could be as simple as "May this day be calm."
- Every time you move through the cycle of baby activities – changing, feeding, sleeping, playing, feeding and so on – find, and focus on, at least one thing that you are grateful for.
- When feeding your baby, intentionally connect with the feeling of their body next to yours, tune into the flow of your breath or perhaps do a short body scan (see page 59) to help really anchor you into the here and now of this precious time with your new baby.

Starter Questions for Journaling After Your Baby Has Been Born

If you like the idea explored in the Introduction of developing a regular mindful journaling practice to help you lean into the experience of each stage of pregnancy and keep a record of it, here are some questions to help you get started:

- You've given birth! What are you feeling most proud of?

- How did it feel to hold your baby for the first time?

- Take a moment to reflect on the environment that your baby has been born into. What season is it? What are the physical surroundings like? Who are the main people in your lives?

- Consider the support you have been receiving from your loved ones since the arrival of your baby. What has been most helpful? And what do you most appreciate about this?

- What are some of your main hopes and dreams for your child?

Feel free to write or draw your answers in any form that naturally emerges; there is no right or wrong here.

Also feel free to ask your own questions and explore your own topics if you want – whether instead of or as well as these ones.

A CLOSING NOTE

Whether you have come to this book new to mindfulness or as someone with an already-established practice, we hope that it has provided you with some gentle, compassionate focus and skills to support you through this unique time of great change.

Babies and young children are naturally mindful, so let your baby become your mindfulness teacher as you grow together. As much as they will learn from you, you will learn from them – and, together, you can thrive.

ACKNOWLEDGEMENTS

I would like to acknowledge the work and dedication of the
Mindfulness in Maternity Team at the Oxford University Hospitals
NHS Foundation Trust. I would also like to extend my gratitude to
the MBCP Midwife Teachers, Annie, Catriona, Kim, Nicki, Penny,
and MBCP Teachers, Eliza and Guin.

I am also grateful for the support of the Oxford Mindfulness
Centre in particular Mark Williams and Maret Dymond, and the
inspiration provided by Nancy Bardacke and the Mindful Birth
and Parenting Foundation.

Sian

USEFUL RESOURCES

Below are some resources for further information and guidance on mindful pregnancy, birthing and parenting in particular, and the practice of mindfulness in general.

BOOKS

Aldort, Naomi, *Raising our Children, Raising Ourselves*, Book Publishers Network, 2006

Bardacke, Nancy, *Mindful Birthing*, HarperOne, 2012

Bogels, Susan, *Mindful Parenting: Finding Space To Be – In a World of To Do,* Pavilion Publishing and Media Ltd, 2020

Dimidjian, Sona and Goodman, Sherryl H., *Expecting Mindfully*, Taylor & Francis Ltd, 2019

Hanh, Thich Nhat, *Planting Seeds: Practicing Mindfulness with Children*, Parallax Press, 2011

Kabat-Zinn, Myla and Jon, *Everyday Blessings: Mindfulness for Parents,* Hyperion, 2011

Puddicombe, Andy, *The Headspace Guide to a Mindful Pregnancy*, Hodder, 2017

Shapiro, Shauna and White, Chris, *Mindful Discipline: A Loving Approach to Setting Limits and Raising an Emotionally Intelligent Child,* New Harbinger Publications, 2014

Williams, Mark and Penman, Danny, *Mindfulness: A Practical Guide to Finding Peace in a Frantic World,* Piatkus Books, 2011

APPS
10% Happier / Buddify / Calm / Frantic World / Headspace / Insight Timer

WEBSITES AND GROUPS
Oxford Mindfulness Centre: oxfordmindfulness.org
Mindful: mindful.org
Headspace: headspace.com
Action for Happiness: actionforhappiness.org
Breathworks: breathworks-mindfulness.org.uk
Mindfulness in Schools Project: mindfulnessinschools.org

REFERENCES

INTRODUCTION

Warriner S, Crane C, Dymond M, Krusche A. An evaluation of mindfulness-based childbirth and parenting courses for pregnant women and prospective fathers/partners within the UK NHS (MBCP-4-NHS). *Midwifery*. 2018; 64:1-10. doi: 10.1016/j.midw.2018.05.004

Newman L, Judd F, Komiti A. Developmental implications of maternal antenatal anxiety mechanisms and approaches to intervention, *Translational Developmental Psychiatry*. 2017; 5:1, doi: 10.1080/20017022.2017.1309879

Sbrilli MD, Duncan LG, Laurent HK. Effects of prenatal mindfulness-based childbirth education on child-bearers' trajectories of distress: a randomized control trial. *BMC Pregnancy Childbirth*. 2020; 20:623. doi: 10.1186/s12884-020-03318-8

Felder JN, Laraia B, Coleman-Phox K, *et al*. Poor sleep quality, psychological distress, and the buffering effect of mindfulness training during pregnancy. *Behav Sleep Med*. 2018; 16(6):611-624. doi: 10.1080/15402002.2016.1266488

CHAPTER 1

Lönnberg G, Nissen E, Niemi M. What is learned from Mindfulness Based Childbirth and Parenting Education? – Participants' experiences. *BMC Pregnancy Childbirth*. 2018; 18(1):466. doi: 10.1186/s12884-018-2098-1

Doll A, Hölzel BK, Mulej Bratec S, *et al*. Mindful attention to breath regulates emotions via increased amygdala-prefrontal cortex connectivity. *Neuroimage*. 2016; 134:305-313. doi: 10.1016/j.neuroimage.2016.03.041

Gentile DA, Sweet DM, He L. Caring for others cares for the self: an experimental test of brief downward social comparison, loving-kindness, and interconnectedness contemplations. *J Happiness Stud*. 2020; 21: 765–778. doi: 10.1007/s10902-019-00100-2

CHAPTER 2

Uvnäs-Moberg K, Handlin L, Petersson M. Self-soothing behaviors with particular reference to oxytocin release induced by non-noxious sensory stimulation. *Front Psychol*. 2015; 5:1529. doi: 10.3389/fpsyg.2014.01529

Uvnäs-Moberg, K, *The Oxytocin Factor: Tapping the Hormone of Calm, Love and Healing*, De Capo Press, 2003

CHAPTER 3

Tang YY, Hölzel BK, Posner MI. The neuroscience of mindfulness meditation. *Nat Rev Neurosci*. 2015; 6(4):213-25. doi: 10.1038/nrn3916

CHAPTER 4

Duncan LG, Cohn MA, Chao MT, *et al*. Benefits of preparing for childbirth with mindfulness training: a randomized controlled trial with active comparison. *BMC Pregnancy Childbirth*. 2017; 17:140. doi: 10.1186/s12884-017-1319-3

CHAPTER 5

Sbrilli MD, Duncan LG, Laurent HK. Effects of prenatal mindfulness-based childbirth education on child-bearers' trajectories of distress: a randomized control trial. *BMC Pregnancy Childbirth*. 2020; 20:623. doi: 10.1186/s12884-020-03318-8

Duncan LG, Coatsworth JD, Greenberg MT. A model of mindful parenting: implications for parent-child relationships and prevention research. *Clin Child Fam Psychol Rev*. 2009; 12(3):255-270. doi: 10.1007/s10567-009-0046-3

TriggerHub.org is one of the most elite and scientifically proven forms of mental health intervention

Trigger Publishing is the leading independent mental health and wellbeing publisher in the UK and US. Clinical and scientific research conducted by assistant professor Dr Kristin Kosyluk and her highly acclaimed team in the Department of Mental Health Law & Policy at the University of South Florida (USF), as well as complementary research by her peers across the US, has independently verified the power of lived experience as a core component in achieving mental health prosperity. Specifically, the lived experiences contained within our bibliotherapeutic books are intrinsic elements in reducing stigma, making those with poor mental health feel less alone, providing the privacy they need to heal, ensuring they know the essential steps to kick-start their own journeys to recovery, and providing hope and inspiration when they need it most.

Delivered through TriggerHub, our unique online portal and accompanying smartphone app, we make our library of bibliotherapeutic titles and other vital resources accessible to individuals and organizations anywhere, at any time and with complete privacy, a crucial element of recovery. As such, TriggerHub is the primary recommendation across the UK and US for the delivery of lived experiences.

At Trigger Publishing and TriggerHub, we proudly lead the way in making the unseen become seen. We are dedicated to humanizing mental health, breaking stigma and challenging outdated societal values to create real action and impact. Find out more about our world-leading work with lived experience and bibliotherapy via triggerhub.org, or by joining us on:

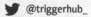 @triggerhub_

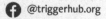 @triggerhub.org

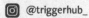 @triggerhub_

Printed in the USA
CPSIA information can be obtained
at www.ICGtesting.com
JSHW031714140824
68134JS00038B/3681

9 781837 962525